Toward a Culture of Consequences

of Consequences

Performance-Based Accountability
Systems for Public Services

Executive Summary

Brian M. Stecher, Frank Camm, Cheryl L. Damberg,
Laura S. Hamilton, Kathleen J. Mullen, Christopher Nelson,
Paul Sorensen, Martin Wachs, Allison Yoh, Gail L. Zellman,
with Kristin J. Leuschner

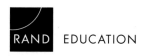

RAND EDUCATION

The research described in this report was conducted within RAND Education, a unit of the RAND Corporation, under a grant from a private philanthropic organization.

Library of Congress Cataloging-in-Publication Data is available for this publication.

ISBN 978-0-8330-5016-8

The RAND Corporation is a nonprofit research organization providing objective analysis and effective solutions that address the challenges facing the public and private sectors around the world. RAND's publications do not necessarily reflect the opinions of its research clients and sponsors.

RAND® is a registered trademark.

Cover image courtesy Fotosearch

Published 2010 by the RAND Corporation
1776 Main Street, P.O. Box 2138, Santa Monica, CA 90407-2138
1200 South Hayes Street, Arlington, VA 22202-5050
4570 Fifth Avenue, Suite 600, Pittsburgh, PA 15213-2665
RAND URL: http://www.rand.org/
To order RAND documents or to obtain additional information, contact
Distribution Services: Telephone: (310) 451-7002;
Fax: (310) 451-6915; Email: order@rand.org

Preface

During the past two decades, performance-based accountability—the application of incentives on the basis of measured outcomes as a means of improving services to the public—has gained popularity in a wide range of public service fields. This document summarizes a monograph that presents the findings of a cross-sector analysis of the effectiveness of performance-based accountability systems (PBASs) for improving public services in child care, education, health care, public health emergency preparedness (PHEP), and transportation. The purpose of the study was to examine the empirical evidence about the use of PBASs in these sectors and to analyze the factors associated with effective PBAS design, implementation, and outcomes.

The monograph and this summary are directed toward decision-makers charged with designing PBASs for public services—typically, committees consisting of government agency directors, consultants, service providers, and researchers—who want to know how to develop and implement a system effectively. The documents should also be of interest to policymakers and their staffs who are charged with deciding whether to adopt a PBAS and why and how to evaluate one.

A companion report presents our analytic framework for describing how a PBAS works and uses the framework to identify appropriate questions to ask when studying the operation and impact of PBASs.[1]

---

[1] Frank Camm and Brian M. Stecher, *Analyzing the Operation of Performance-Based Accountability Systems for Public Services*, Santa Monica, Calif.: RAND Corporation, TR-853, 2010. As of August 2010: http://www.rand.org/pubs/technical_reports/TR853/

This research was undertaken within RAND Education, a unit of the RAND Corporation. Funding to conduct the study was provided by a private, philanthropic organization.

Questions and comments about this summary should be directed to the authors:

Brian Stecher
1776 Main Street
P.O. Box 2138
Santa Monica, CA 90407-2138
Tel: (310) 393-0411 x6579
Fax: (310) 393-4818
Brian_Stecher@rand.org

Frank Camm
1200 South Hayes Street
Arlington, VA 22202-5050
Tel: (703) 413-1100 x5261
Fax: (703) 413-8111
Frank_Camm@rand.org

More information about RAND Education is available at http://www.rand.org/education/.

Contents

Table

Acknowledgments

A number of individuals made important contributions to the work described in the monograph. Sylvia Montoya conducted a literature review that we used to provide background information and to frame the discussions of accountability in each sector. In addition, participants at a 2008 workshop reacted to our early thinking about PBASs, providing helpful, critical feedback and offering new perspectives on our work. These participants included Dominic Brewer, University of Southern California; Jon Christianson, University of Minnesota; Carl Cohn, Claremont Graduate University; William Gormley Jr., Georgetown University; LeRoy Graymer, University of California, Los Angeles (UCLA), Extension; Jayetta Hecker, U.S. Government Accountability Office; Joan Herman, UCLA; Sylvia Hysong, Baylor College of Medicine; Richard Little, University of Southern California; Betsey Lyman, California Department of Public Health; Kathy Malaske-Samu, Los Angeles County Office of Child Care; Meera Mani, Preschool California; Steven Pickrell, Cambridge Systematics; Nico Potterat, Los Angeles Health Care Plan; Gery Ryan, RAND Corporation; Linda Smith, National Association for Child Care Resource and Referral Agencies; Joan Sollenberger, California Department of Transportation; Donna Spiker, SRI International; Sam Stebbins, University of Pittsburgh; Mark Steinmeyer, Smith Richardson Foundation; Michael Stoto, Georgetown University; Fred Tempes, WestEd; and Craig Thomas, Centers for Disease Control and Prevention. Donna White expertly coordinated the workshop and provided invaluable administrative assistance on other aspects of this project.

The quality of this document was substantially improved through several stages of review. Our RAND colleague Richard Neu reviewed an early draft of the monograph and provided constructive suggestions that led to important changes. We are also grateful to William Gormley and Harry Hatry, who served as our formal peer reviewers, and to Cathy Stasz, RAND Education Quality Assurance Manager, for their thoughtful reviews.

Abbreviations

A+B	cost plus time
CAA	Clean Air Act of 1963
CAFE	Corporate Average Fuel Economy
CDC	Centers for Disease Control and Prevention
CMS	Centers for Medicare and Medicaid Services
EPA	U.S. Environmental Protection Agency
EPCA	Energy Policy and Conservation Act
FTA	Federal Transit Administration
HEDIS	Healthcare Effectiveness Data and Information Set
HHS	U.S. Department of Health and Human Services
HMO	health maintenance organization
mpg	miles per gallon
NACCHO	National Association of County and City Health Officials
NCLB	No Child Left Behind Act of 2001
NCQA	National Committee for Quality Assurance
NTD	National Transit Database

P4P   pay for performance

P4R   pay for reporting

PAHPA   Pandemic and All-Hazards Preparedness Act

PBAS   performance-based accountability system

PHEP   public health emergency preparedness

QRIS   quality rating and improvement system

SBR   standards-based reform

SIP   state implementation plan

SUV   sport-utility vehicle

Executive Summary

During the past two decades, PBASs, which link financial or other incentives to measured performance as a means of improving services to the public, have gained popularity in a wide range of service fields. There are many examples. In education, the No Child Left Behind Act of 2001 (NCLB)[2] combined explicit expectations for student performance with well-aligned tests to measure achievement and strong consequences for schools that do not meet program targets. In child care, quality rating and improvement systems (QRISs) establish quality standards, measure and rate providers, and provide incentives and supports for quality improvement. In the transportation sector, cost-plus-time (A+B) contracting is used to streamline highway construction; in health care, there are more than 40 hospitals and more than 100 physician and medical group performance-based accountability (popularly dubbed pay-for-performance, or P4P) programs in place in the United States. There have also been recent efforts to create performance measures and establish consequences related to the nation's efforts to prevent, protect against, respond to, and recover from large-scale public health emergencies.

While PBASs can vary widely across sectors, they share three main components: goals (i.e., one or more long-term outcomes to be achieved), incentives (i.e., rewards or sanctions to motivate changes in individual or organizational behavior to improve performance), and

---

[2] Public Law 107-110, No Child Left Behind Act of 2001, January 8, 2002. As of June 7, 2010: http://frwebgate.access.gpo.gov/cgi-bin/getdoc.cgi?dbname=107_cong_public_laws&docid=f:publ110.107.pdf

measures (formal mechanisms for monitoring the delivery of services or the attainment of goals).

Today's PBASs grew out of efforts over many years and many countries to manage the private and public organizations that were growing too large to be overseen by a single manager who knew what everyone was doing. These innovative approaches focused on measuring *performance*, which was originally defined fairly narrowly. Over time, notions about what aspects of performance most mattered broadened and changed. By the 1980s, government organizations were linking performance to incentives in an effort to motivate and direct individual performance and improve organizational outcomes.

But while the use of PBASs has spread in the public sector, little is known about whether such programs are having the desired effect. Research suggests that PBASs influence provider behaviors, a first step toward achieving outcomes, but there is currently little evidence concerning the effectiveness of PBASs at achieving their performance goals, or the experiences of governments and agencies at the forefront of this trend. The monograph seeks to address the gap by examining several examples of PBASs, large and small, in a range of public service areas. This study examines nine PBASs that are drawn from five sectors: child care, education, health care, PHEP, and transportation (Table S.1). The cases we studied provide useful information on the formation, design, operation, and evaluation of PBASs.

The choice of cases was guided by practical as well as theoretical considerations. On the practical side, we wanted to take advantage of the expertise available at RAND, where empirical research is being conducted on a number of performance measurement and accountability systems in different service areas. On the theoretical side, we wanted to include cases in which services are provided primarily by public agencies (education, transportation), as well as sectors in which services are provided primarily by private organizations but in which the public sector has an important role in governance (child care, health care). We also wanted to include at least one instance in which measurement itself was a challenge (PHEP).

Table S.1
Cases Examined in This Study

Sector	PBAS	Key Incentive
Child care	QRISs	Prestige associated with high rating Financial incentives
Education	NCLB	Graduated set of interventions regarding professional development, instruction, staffing, and school governance (e.g., constraints on use of funds)
	P4P	Cash bonuses, salary increases
Health care	Hospital and physician or medical group P4P programs, including quality "report cards"	Financial payments for high performance or improvement, public recognition, transparency (i.e., clarity and openness) of performance results
PHEP	CDC PHEP cooperative agreement	Withholding of federal funds for failure to meet performance benchmarks
Transportation	A+B highway construction contracting	Financial rewards or sanctions based on time to complete
	CAFE standards	Fines for failure to meet minimum average fuel-efficiency standards
	CAA ambient air pollution conformity requirements	Federal transportation funds subject to conformity with ambient air quality standards
	Transit subsidy allocation formulas	Share of state or regional funding for local transit operators

NOTE: CDC = Centers for Disease Control and Prevention. CAFE = Corporate Average Fuel Economy. CAA = Clean Air Act (Public Law 88-206, Clean Air Act of 1963, December 17, 1963, and its amendments).

Research Approach

The research approach included a broad review of literature related to performance measurement and accountability, the development of an analytic framework to structure our internal discussions about research evidence in the five sectors, a 1.5-day integrative workshop that examined various features of PBASs (e.g., context in which the PBAS arose, measures, incentives, and evaluation approaches), and analysis of sector-specific empirical results and identification of cross-sector principles. Through this process, we attempted to derive principles that might have general applicability beyond the cases we studied.

Findings

Evidence on the effects of nine PBASs in five sectors shows that, under the right circumstances, a PBAS can be an effective strategy for improving the delivery of services to the public. Optimum circumstances include having the following:

- a goal that is widely shared
- measures that are unambiguous and easy to observe
- incentives that apply to individuals or organizations that have control over the relevant inputs and processes
- incentives that are meaningful to those being incentivized
- few competing interests or requirements
- adequate resources to design, implement, and operate the PBAS.

However, these conditions are rarely fully realized, so it is difficult to design and implement PBASs that are uniformly effective. The following sections highlight the major factors that influence PBAS development and effects in the cases we studied.

Decision to Adopt a Performance-Based Accountability System Is Shaped by Political, Historical, and Cultural Contexts

In the cases we examined, the decision to adopt a PBAS was subject to multiple influences. In many sectors, the process was heavily influenced by the preferences of service providers—the very people whose behavior the PBAS sought to shape. In transportation, for instance, PBASs designed to improve local transit funding have often been strongly influenced by the local jurisdictions that are the subject of the PBASs. Given conflicts among stakeholders, it is perhaps not surprising that PBASs often proceed in spite of a lack of clear agreement on what constitutes performance and on who should be held accountable for what. In many sectors, there is not a sufficiently strong evidence base to provide scientific guidance to would-be PBAS adopters and designers.

The creation of PBASs might be nurtured by the presence of a strong history and culture of performance measurement and accountability. In education, for instance, measurement of student performance has a long history in the United States, and standardized achievement tests are accepted as an indicator of performance for many purposes. However, such a history does not ensure the smooth adoption of a PBAS. Many PBASs, once created, exist in conflict with other PBASs and governance structures. This is especially the case in sectors with a long tradition of measurement and accountability in which service providers receive funds from multiple sources and through many funding mechanisms (e.g., transportation, health care, education).

Selection of Incentive Structures Has Proven Challenging

PBAS designers face three basic design issues:

- determining whose behavior they seek to change (i.e., identifying individuals or organizations to target)
- deciding on the type and size of incentives
- measuring performance and linking these measures to the incentives they have chosen.

In the PBASs we examined, it was fairly easy in most cases to identify the individuals or organizations that are held accountable for improving service activities and reaching the PBAS goals. It has been more challenging, however, to decide which incentive structures to use to affect the desired behaviors.

Context can have a large effect on the incentive structures that PBAS designers choose. For example, when participation in a PBAS is voluntary, designers of PBASs typically use rewards rather than sanctions. We found that, when the designers of a PBAS worked within a regulatory setting (e.g., NCLB, PHEP), sanctions were more common. In contrast, designers of PBASs in which participation was voluntary—child care and A+B contracting, for example—tended to prefer rewards. The size and details of rewards vary widely across the PBASs we studied. It is unclear how well the magnitude of rewards is correlated with the benefits of the changes that the PBAS designers seek to induce or the effort that service providers, such as doctors and teachers, must make to comply with these changes.

Design of Performance Measures Requires a Balance Among Competing Priorities

The measures used to quantify performance can vary in many dimensions. PBAS designers must consider a number of competing factors when selecting and structuring measures:

- the feasibility, availability, and cost of measures
- the context within which a PBAS operates
- the alignment of measures with PBAS goals
- the degree of control of the monitored party
- resistance to manipulation by the monitored service activity
- understandability.

The selection of performance measures ultimately requires some trade-offs among these factors. PBAS designers seem to prefer measures that can be collected at low cost or that already exist outside the PBAS. To choose among potentially acceptable measures, a PBAS tends to balance two major considerations: the alignment of a measure with the PBAS's goals and the extent to which the individuals or organizations monitored by the PBAS have the ability to control the value of that measure. A natural tension arises from efforts to achieve balance between these objectives. Over time, the parties that a PBAS monitors might find ways to "game" the system, increasing their standing on a measure in ways that are not aligned with the PBAS goals. Perhaps the best-known example of such manipulation in the cases we examined is the act of "teaching to the test" in an educational setting.

Continuing vigilance and flexibility can help a PBAS manage this tension and maintain the balance between policymakers' priorities and the capabilities of the parties the PBAS monitors. Such a balance tends to be easier to achieve when the measures the PBAS uses are understandable and have been communicated to all parties.

Successful Implementation Must Overcome Many Potential Pitfalls

Even a well-designed PBAS might not yield the desired results if it is not executed effectively. Our review of the literature and the nine cases identified several pitfalls that can occur on the implementation process:

- lack of PBAS experience and infrastructure
- unrealistic timelines
- complexity of the PBAS
- failure to communicate
- stakeholder resistance.

There are many strategies available to address these pitfalls. For example, when building a PBAS, exploiting the existing infrastructure, when possible, and implementing in stages can minimize both the time needed for implementation and the disruptive potential of mistakes before they can compound. Incorporating a pilot-testing phase can also head off a number of problems early. Communicating with stakeholders is also integral to the success of the PBAS, while formative monitoring can be important for identifying and correcting problems that occur during implementation.

Evidence of System Effectiveness Is Limited and Leads to Varying Conclusions by Sector

In general, PBASs have not been subject to rigorous evaluation, and the evidence that does exist leads to somewhat different conclusions by sector:

- In education, it is clear that NCLB and other high-stakes testing programs with public reporting and other incentives at the school level have led to changes in teacher behavior; however, teachers seem to respond narrowly in ways that improve measured outputs (i.e., the measures) with less attention to long-term outcomes (i.e., the goals).[3] While student test scores have risen, there is uncertainty as to whether these reflect more learning or are to some degree the product of teaching to the test or other approaches to generating apparent improvement.

- In health care, relatively small financial incentives (frequently combined with public reporting) have had some modest effects in improving the quality of care delivered.
- Examples from the transportation sector suggest that large financial incentives can lead to creative solutions, as well as to lobbying to influence the demands of the PBAS regulation. The latter has been the case with the CAFE standards, which require automobile manufacturers to achieve a minimum level of fuel economy for the fleet of vehicles sold each year in the United States.
- It is too soon to judge the effectiveness of PBASs in child care and PHEP.

PBASs also have the potential to cause unintended consequences by incentivizing the wrong kind of behavior or encouraging undesirable effects. For example, in NCLB, attaching public reporting and other incentives to test scores has led to unintended behavioral changes (i.e., teaching to the test) that might be considered undesirable. In the transportation sector, some analysts have argued that CAFE standards prompted auto manufacturers to produce smaller and lighter vehicles, which, in turn, increased the number of crash-related injuries and fatal-

---

[3] We use the following terminology when talking about public service programs and their consequences: a program is a structured activity that transforms *inputs* into *outputs*, which are observable, measurable (e.g., blood pressure, test scores, parts per million of carbon dioxide, or CO_2), and easy to associate directly with the program. Ultimately, these outputs affect long-term *outcomes* that are of interest to policymakers (health, achievement, air quality). The outcomes might or might not be measurable, but it is typically difficult to draw a direct connection between the program and these outcomes. Many factors beyond the program's control or even understanding might affect the relationship between the program and the higher-level, broad outcomes relevant to policymakers. As a result, to influence behavior within a program with confidence, an accountability system must focus on measures of *outputs* that can be clearly attributed to the program.

ities, though this conclusion remains subject to some debate. A concern in the health-care sector is that PBASs include a narrow set of performance markers, which might increase physicians' focus on what is measured and reduce their attention to unmeasured effects. However, to date, there is an absence of empirical evidence showing such effects.

If a PBAS does not initially meet its aims, it does not mean that a PBAS cannot be successful; it might just mean that some of the structural details require further refinement. PBASs are sufficiently complex that initial success is rare, and the need for modification should be anticipated.

Recommendations for System Developers

We offer a number of recommendations for PBAS sponsors, designers, and other stakeholders to consider regarding PBAS design, incentives and performance measurement, implementation, and evaluation.

Design of the Performance-Based Accountability System

Designing a PBAS is a complex undertaking, and many of the decisions that will need to be made are heavily dependent on sector-specific contextual circumstances.

Consider the Factors That Might Hinder or Support the Success of a PBAS to See Whether Conditions Support Its Use. The first issue is to consider whether a PBAS is the best policy approach for the policy concern at hand and whether it might be expected to succeed. From the cases examined, we identified a number of factors that tend to support a successful PBAS implementation:

- broad agreement on the nature of the problem
- broad agreement on PBAS goals
- knowledge that specific changes in inputs, structures, processes, or outputs will lead to improved outcomes
- ability of service providers, through changes in behavior, to exert significant influence on outputs and outcomes

- ability of the implementing organization to modify the incentive structure for service providers
- absence of competing programs that send conflicting signals to service providers
- political context in which it is acceptable for the PBAS to be gradually improved over time
- sufficient resources to create the PBAS and to respond to the incentives.

If a large share of these factors does not hold for the application under consideration, decisionmakers might wish to consider alternative policy options or think about ways to influence the context to create more-positive conditions for a PBAS.

Be Sensitive to the Context for Implementation. It is important to account for constraints and leverage opportunities presented by the context in which the PBAS will be implemented. Such considerations include the extent to which the implementing organization can alter the incentive structure faced by service providers, existing mechanisms that will affect the behavior of service providers (e.g., safety or licensing requirements) or that can be used to support the PBAS (e.g., data collection), and current knowledge of the service activity covered by the PBAS.

Consider Applying Performance Measures and Incentives at Different Functional Levels. If the service-delivery activities are organized hierarchically (e.g., students within classrooms within schools within districts), PBAS designers should consider the application of performance measures and incentives at different functional levels within the activity (e.g., different measures and incentives for school districts, school principals, and teachers or for hospitals, clinics, and doctors). Provided that the performance measures and incentives are structured in a complementary fashion, the results can be additive and mutually reinforcing.

Design the PBAS So That It Can Be Monitored Over Time. To obtain the best results over the long term, it is important to develop a plan for monitoring the PBAS, identifying shortcomings that might be limiting the effectiveness of the PBAS or leading to unintended consequences, and modifying the program as needed.

Incentives and Performance Measurement

The selection of incentives and performance measures is of vital importance to the PBAS. The type and magnitude of the incentives will govern the level of effort providers expend to influence the performance measures, while the measures will dictate the things on which the service providers should focus and what they might choose to ignore or neglect.

Create an Incentive Structure Compatible with the Culture of the Service Activity. Many options for incentives are available, including cash, promotions, status, recognition, increased autonomy, or access to training or other investment resources. The goal is to select options that will best influence behavior without undermining intrinsic service motivation.

Make the Rewards or Penalties Big Enough to Matter. The size of the incentive should outweigh the effort required by the service provider to improve on the performance measure; otherwise, service providers will simply not make the effort. However, the size of the incentives should not exceed the value obtained from improved provider behavior, since the PBAS would, by definition, not be cost-effective.

Focus on Performance Measures That Matter. Performance measures determine how service providers focus their efforts. To the extent possible, therefore, it makes sense to include those measures believed to have the greatest effect on the broader goals of interest.

Create Measures That Treat Service Providers Fairly. In certain settings, the ability of service providers to influence desired outputs might be limited. When selecting performance measures, PBAS developers should consider the degree to which service providers can influence the criteria of interest. Individuals or organizations should not be held accountable for things they do not control. In such cases, there are other options for creating performance measures that treat service providers fairly:

- Create "risk-adjusted" output measures that account for relevant social, physical, and demographic characteristics of the population served.
- Establish measures based on inputs, structure, or processes rather than on outputs or outcomes.
- Measure relative improvement rather than absolute performance.

Avoid Measures That Focus on a Single Absolute Threshold Score. Although the threshold approach can be intuitively appealing (in the sense that the specified score represents a quality bar that all service providers should strive to achieve), in practice, measures that focus on a single threshold can prove quite problematic. Low achievers with no realistic prospects for achieving the absolute threshold score will have no incentive to seek even modest improvements, while high achievers will have no incentive to strive for further improvement. Alternatives include use of multithreshold scores and measurement of year-over-year improvement.

Implementation

It is possible to create a potentially effective design for a PBAS and then fail to implement the design successfully; thus, special attention needs to be paid to the way the PBAS is implemented.

Implement the Program in Stages. Because most PBASs are quite complex, it is often helpful to develop and introduce different components in sequence, modifying as needed in response to any issues that arise. For example, initial efforts and funding might focus on the development of capacity to measure and report performance, with measures and incentives rolled out over time. Pilot-testing might also be used to assess measures and other design features.

Integrate the PBAS with Existing Performance Databases and Accounting and Personnel Systems. A PBAS is not created in a void; rather, it must be incorporated within existing structures and systems. It is thus important to think through all of the ways in which the PBAS will need to interact with preexisting infrastructure—e.g., performance databases, accounting systems, and personnel systems. These considerations might suggest changes in the design of the PBAS or highlight ways in which the existing infrastructure needs to be modified while the PBAS is being created.

Engage Providers, and, to the Extent Possible, Secure Their Support. To garner the support of providers, it is helpful to develop measures that are credible (i.e., tied to outcomes about which they care), fair (i.e., that account for external circumstances beyond the control of providers), and actionable (i.e., that can be positively influenced through appropriate actions by the service provider). A good approach is to involve providers in the process of developing the measures and incentives. While, to some degree, it can be expected that service providers will seek to weaken the targets or standards to their benefit, those responsible for implementing and overseeing the PBAS will need to judge whether lowering performance expectations would ultimately undermine the success of the PBAS.

Ensure That Providers and Other Stakeholders Understand Measures and Incentives. Communication is key. Particularly in cases in which there are numerous providers with varying internal support systems to enable engagement—as, for example, with health-care P4P systems and child-care quality ratings—it can be helpful to employ multiple communications channels (e.g., email, website, conference presentations) as appropriate.

Plan for the Likelihood That Certain Measures Will "Top Out." As service providers improve their performance in response to the incentive structure, a growing percentage might achieve the highest possible scores for certain measures. PBAS designers should plan for this eventuality, e.g., by replacing topped-out measures with more-challenging ones or by requiring service providers to maintain a high level of performance for topped-out measures in order to qualify for incentives.

Provide Resources to Support Provider Improvement. It can be valuable to devote program resources to support efforts at improvement. This might involve infrastructure investments or education for providers on becoming more effective.

Evaluation

Ironically, given the spirit of accountability embodied in the PBAS approach, most of the cases reviewed in this study have not been subjected to rigorous evaluation. We believe that it is vitally important to rectify this lack of evaluation. Only through careful monitoring and evaluation can decisionmakers detect problems and take steps to improve the functioning of the PBAS over time.

Consider Using a Third Party to Evaluate the PBAS. Not all organizations that implement a PBAS possess the necessary methodological expertise to conduct a sound programmatic evaluation. Additionally, many implementing organizations, for understandable reasons, will tend to be biased in favor of positive results. For these reasons, it is beneficial to rely on an independent and qualified third party to conduct an evaluation of the PBAS.

Structure the Evaluation of a PBAS Based on Its Stage of Development. When a system is first developed, it might be most helpful to evaluate implementation activities (e.g., whether appropriate mechanisms for capturing and reporting performance measures have been developed). As the system matures, the focus should shift to evaluating the effects, in terms of observed provider behavior and service outputs, of the performance measures and incentive structure. An evaluation should focus on outputs only after performance measures and incentives have been in place long enough to influence behavior.

Examine the Effects of the PBAS on Both Procedures and Outputs. One approach for doing so is to develop a logic model, a visual representation of the ways in which the PBAS is intended to influence provider behavior. This model can then become the basis for thoughtful monitoring and evaluation and make it easier to plan the evaluation of a PBAS based on its stage of development.

Use the Strongest Possible Research Design Given the Context in Which the PBAS Exists. Options, sorted in order of decreasing rigor, include randomized control trials, regression discontinuity designs, nonequivalent-group designs, lagged implementation designs, and case studies. If certain design aspects are flexible, it might be possible to implement variations in the PBAS coupled with common evaluation frameworks to provide rigorous comparison and help choose the most effective options. Such variations could include different performance measures, different types of incentives, or different incentive levels (e.g., significant versus modest financial rewards).

Implement Additional, Nonincentivized Measures to Verify Improvement and Test for Unintended Consequences. A PBAS might induce service-provider responses that lead to improved performance scores without corresponding improvement in the underlying objectives (e.g., a teacher might invest instructional effort on test-taking strategies that lead to improvement on standardized test scores that overstates actual student gains in mastery of the broader subject matter). To detect when this might be occurring, it can be helpful to include nonincentivized measures intended to test similar concepts (e.g., additional math and reading exams in alternative test formats to check whether there has been a comparable level of improvement). Nonincentivized measures can also be used to examine whether a focus on the incentivized measures within the PBAS is causing other areas of performance to be neglected.

Link the PBAS Evaluation to a Review and Redesign Process. The true benefits of evaluation come not from simply understanding what is working and what is not, but rather from applying that understanding to improve the functioning of the PBAS. Evaluation should thus be embedded within a broader framework for monitoring and continuing to refine the PBAS over time.

Areas for Further Research

Because so few of the PBASs that we examined have been subjected to rigorous testing and evaluation, there are a number of fundamental questions that our study cannot answer about the design, implementation, and performance of PBASs. Policymakers would benefit from research—both within individual sectors and across sectors—on the short- and long-term impact of PBASs, the elements of a PBAS that are most important in determining its effectiveness, and the cost and cost-effectiveness of PBASs, particularly in comparison to other policy approaches.

Concluding Thoughts

This study suggests that PBASs represent a promising policy option for improving the quality of service-delivery activities in many contexts. The evidence supports continued experimentation with and adoption of this approach in appropriate circumstances. Even so, the appropriate design for a PBAS and, ultimately, its prospects for success are highly dependent on the context in which it will operate. Because PBASs are typically complex, getting all of the details right with the initial implementation is rare.

Ongoing system evaluation and monitoring should be viewed, to a far greater extent than in prior efforts, as an integral component of the PBAS. Evaluation and monitoring provide the necessary information to refine and improve the functioning of the system over time. Additionally, more-thorough evaluation and monitoring of PBASs will lead, gradually, to a richer evidence base that should help future decisionmakers understand (1) the circumstances under which a PBAS would be an effective and cost-effective policy instrument and (2) the most appropriate design features to employ when developing a PBAS for a given set of circumstances.

The Five Sectors

This appendix provides a brief description of each of the sectors and the relevant PBASs covered in the monograph. The descriptions are based on our knowledge and research expertise.

Child Care

Child care is funded and delivered by public agencies at all levels of government and a variety of private organizations as part of what has been described as a "non-system of micro-enterprises."[1] Formal child-care programs operate in a range of settings, including free-standing centers, public school campuses, churches, community centers, and family homes. Program models include full-day care for ages 0–5, pre-K programs for four-year-olds (and, in some states, three-year-olds), and part-day preschool programs. Programs might be funded entirely by parent fees or federal monies, receive subsidies for children whose families qualify, receive in-kind subsidies from the churches or other organizations that sponsor and house them, or rely mainly on parent volunteers as part of child-care cooperatives. Child care is an imperfect market in several respects: (1) Programs are generally underfunded because most parents cannot afford to pay the full cost of care and public subsidies are set at less than full cost; (2) the supply of affordable

---

[1] L. S. Kagan, "Buckets, Banks, and Hearts: Aligning Early Childhood Standards and Systems," presentation, Quality Rating and Improvement Systems: Creating the Next Generation of QRISs conference, St. Paul, Minn., June 4, 2008.

care in most areas is limited; and (3) most parents are grateful to find an affordable place for their child that accommodates their work hours.

Although studies have consistently found that average child-care quality is mediocre, the sector has not focused much attention on program quality. Until quite recently, quality standards were largely defined by state licensing requirements, which represented a fairly low bar. Licensing is focused primarily on the adequacy and safety of a program's physical environment, including fencing, square footage, and protection of children's well-being (i.e., are electrical plugs covered? Are cleaning supplies locked up?).

The growing policy attention on K–12 accountability has raised questions about child-care outcomes, particularly school readiness. These questions have led the sector to focus on quality and devise ways to improve it. QRISs represent the most popular current approach to doing so. QRISs produce a single, easy-to-understand rating for each provider, much like restaurant ratings in some cities; QRISs differ from other PBASs in that participation is voluntary. QRISs define quality standards and measure and rate providers, thus making program quality transparent, and provide incentives and supports for quality improvement. Ideally, these systems promote awareness of quality and encourage programs to engage in a process of continuous quality improvement. While QRISs ultimately are expected to promote improved child outcomes, such as increased school readiness, QRISs focus primarily on assessing and improving program inputs and processes. States have found QRISs an attractive approach to improving child-care quality; 19 states now operate QRISs, and several others are developing them.

The rating process and the ratings that result are the major QRIS monitoring activities. Rating systems essentially define child-care quality by identifying which program components will be assessed. States generally measure child-staff ratios, group size, staff education and training, and some indicator of the classroom environment. States differ in whether to include and how to weight parent involvement, national accreditation, and management processes. A number of issues surround QRIS ratings. A key one is integrity: Most measures were designed for low-stakes use, but QRISs are high-stakes systems; summary ratings might affect both program funding and enrollments. Ratings are also quite costly; they typically require hours-long classroom observations. How the different component measures are combined into a single program rating has received no empirical attention.

Early on, one of the key incentives was the prestige associated with a high rating. But significant funds are required to support key quality improvements, such as reduced child-staff ratios and improved staff education and training. As a result, most QRISs now provide financial incentives to support improvements and motivate providers to participate in rating systems. Incentives are generally linked to the summary rating: Higher-rated programs receive more funds to support their higher-quality programs. In higher-stakes QRISs, rating might also affect the level of funding provided for subsidy-eligible children. Many states also provide staff-level incentives, including scholarships or other professional development programs; eligibility generally requires a program rating that denotes at least reasonable quality.

Incentives might also occur in the form of hands-on quality-improvement support. Often, this support begins with detailed feedback on rating results and a specific quality-improvement plan. In many systems, coaches provide specific technical assistance. This package of supports can be very motivating for providers, who often do not know how best to spend the limited quality-improvement funds they receive through their participation in the QRIS process or how to initiate quality-improvement efforts.

Research on QRISs has been limited in both focus and depth. Most efforts focus on testing the validity of these systems and ask basic questions appropriate to this task: Do summary ratings relate to other measures of quality? Are the quality-improvement efforts resulting in improvements in participating-provider quality? A large share of the evaluation studies has focused on examining correlations between environmental ratings and overall program ratings. Typically, moderate correlations are found. Several studies have examined whether average ratings improve over time; generally, they do. However, we do not know how well QRISs measure what they purport to measure or whether children benefit from the improved care they receive as their providers receive quality-improvement support. Many of the measures used to assess the components were developed in low-stakes settings, such as research studies or self-assessments, in which there were few, if any, consequences attached to a particular score. These measures might not be appropriate in high-stakes settings, in which summary ratings could substantially affect a program's bottom line.

Education

Public education in the United States is primarily the responsibility of state and local governments. Traditionally, states reserve for themselves the functions of school accreditation, teacher certification, curriculum adoption, and financial auditing, and states delegate to local districts the responsibility for operations, instructional materials, and staff supervision (although there is considerable variation in this pattern). Districts, in turn, delegate many operational decisions to individual schools. The educational governance system has been described as "loosely coupled" because responsibility is distributed across levels without rigid monitoring and accountability.[2] In most districts, teacher and principal salaries are determined by a negotiated schedule that rewards postsecondary education and job experience but not individual performance.

Until recently, the federal role in public K–12 education has been limited to regulations and supplemental funding designed to promote equity for economically disadvantaged students and students with disabilities. The federal government contributes about 10 percent of the total cost of K–12 education.

In the 1980s and 1990s, some states began to adopt standards-based reforms (SBRs), which were designed to shift the focus of governance from inputs (finance, accreditation, certification) to outputs (student achievement) and to align the elements of the educational system to foster higher achievement. In 2001, this idea was incorporated into federal legislation (NCLB), which is essentially a PBAS that uses schools and districts as the units of accountability. NCLB requires

---

[2]   Karl E. Weick, "Educational Organizations as Loosely Coupled Systems," *Administrative Science Quarterly*, Vol. 21, No. 1, March 1976, pp. 1–9.

that all states create accountability systems that include state standards in reading, mathematics, and science and annual testing of students in selected grades in these subjects.

A second form of PBAS (P4P) is being adopted in some districts and states. P4P systems usually pay bonuses directly to teachers or principals for meeting specific performance criteria, usually in terms of student achievement but, in some cases, including other outputs relevant to students (such as graduation) or educators' practices.

Under NCLB, each state must identify students who are proficient based on reading and mathematics tests. The percentage of students who are proficient in reading and mathematics in each school is compared to a target value, which must increase to 100 percent by 2014. The calculation must be made for the school as a whole and for each significant subgroup of students, including the major racial and ethnic groups, students of low socioeconomic status, English-language learners, and special education students.

Most P4P programs also use the state tests as their primary measure and compute some form of value-added metric to try to determine how much growth is associated with a particular teacher or principal each year.

NCLB includes a graduated set of interventions that are intended to motivate better performance and effect specific changes while also providing schools with needed assistance. P4P systems tend to focus more on rewards than on sanctions, offering cash bonuses (or sometimes salary increases) to teachers and principals whose students meet the performance targets. Some of these systems are competitions, with the highest-performing teachers receiving bonuses, whereas others set fixed growth targets and pay bonuses to any teacher or principal reaching the target.

A large body of research indicates that high-stakes testing has a strong effect on teaching practice.[3] Teachers tend to align their lessons

---

[3] See, e.g., Brian M. Stecher, "Consequences of Large-Scale, High-Stakes Testing on School and Classroom Practices," in Laura S. Hamilton, Brian M. Stecher, and Stephen P. Klein, eds., *Making Sense of Test-Based Accountability in Education*, Santa Monica, Calif.: RAND Corporation, MR-1554-EDU, 2002, pp. 79–100. As of June 6, 2010: http://www.rand.org/pubs/monograph_reports/MR1554/

with both standards and assessments, which often leads to a reduction in time spent on topics and subjects that are not tested. This focus on tested material can lead to *score inflation*, which refers to gains on a test that do not generalize to other measures of the same topic or subject. Some research suggests that, when performance is measured according to a single threshold, such as proficiency, teachers tend to focus on students near that threshold (often called bubble kids). Furthermore, there is some evidence that high stakes lead to excessive test preparation (i.e., practice with specific formats, such as multiple choice) and even cheating.

The literature on P4P is also mixed; some programs have been associated with improvements in achievement, but it is not always possible to distinguish real gains from score inflation. In addition, there is some evidence that teachers and administrators have trouble understanding the information on performance gains reported as value-added measures and that, in some systems, teachers believe that the P4P program has led to negative effects in their schools.

The impact of NCLB and other SBR policies on achievement is uncertain; while scores have increased in many places, it is difficult to know whether these are real gains or stem from score inflation. NCLB appears to have had beneficial effects of focusing attention on student outcomes and highlighting the performance of traditionally low-performing subgroups of students. However, there are no studies of the overall costs and benefits of NCLB or P4P in education. Although only a small percentage of educational spending goes for NCLB accountability provisions, many states have reacted negatively to the accountability requirements and characterized them as unfunded mandates. Some states lack capacity to create and manage high-quality, test-based accountability programs and address the needs of identified schools.

Health Care

Unlike most of the other sectors represented here, health care in the United States is provided primarily by the private sector. Only a quarter of the population is covered by public health insurance (i.e., the elderly and low-income, by Medicare and Medicaid, respectively). In contrast, 60 percent are covered by private health insurance plans. (Roughly 15 percent have no health insurance coverage and typically rely on emergency services.) Most private plans are employer-sponsored, managed care plans. That is, care is based around a network of preferred providers offering lower-cost and more-comprehensive benefits than out-of-network providers. (In the case of health-maintenance organizations, or HMOs, out-of-network care is restricted altogether.)

Performance measurement in health care was initially used internally for quality improvement, but, with the 1990s expansion of managed care, it grew into a mechanism to hold plans accountable. The National Committee for Quality Assurance (NCQA) provides accreditation of health plans and has developed the Healthcare Effectiveness Data and Information Set (HEDIS) to provide plan-quality information to employers. In addition, health plans, employers, consumer advocacy groups, and various government agencies publish quality report cards to assist individuals in choosing their health-care providers (at the level of health plans, medical groups and hospitals or individual physicians). Regardless of these efforts, a 2003 RAND study[4] found that adults in the United States receive only 50 percent of recommended care on average. Currently, most health-care providers are reimbursed regardless of how well they provide care or how efficiently they use resources.

Despite this emphasis on the private sector, Centers for Medicare and Medicaid Services (CMS) remains the dominant purchaser in the market for health-care services because use is much greater in the senior population. (Even though seniors represent only a fraction of the total market, they represent a far greater share of overall health spending.) As a result, any reform to physician or hospital reimbursement under Medicare will have repercussions for the rest of the health sector. While performance-based accountability was initiated in the private

---

[4] Elizabeth A. McGlynn, Steven M. Asch, John Adams, Joan Keesey, Jennifer Hicks, Alison DeCristofaro, and Eve A. Kerr, "The Quality of Health Care Delivered to Adults in the United States," *New England Journal of Medicine*, Vol. 348, No. 26, June 26, 2003, pp. 2635–2645.

sector, pay-for-reporting (P4R) legislation in 2003 and 2006[5] has set the stage for performance-based accountability to move into the public sector through Medicare.

At last count, there were more than 40 hospitals and more than 100 physician and medical-group performance-based accountability (P4P) programs in place in the private sector in the United States. Additionally, CMS is staging a number of P4P demonstrations targeted at hospitals, physician group practices, end-stage renal-disease facilities, nursing homes, and home health workers. Outside the United States, in 2004, the UK's National Health Service rolled out a large-scale P4P program for general practitioners. No single approach to P4P is being used, and there is a wide variation in program designs.

The number and set of measures used in the PBAS programs vary widely from only a few (typically no more than five to ten in the small-scale U.S. programs) to many (e.g., 146 in the case of the UK). The measures are centered primarily on quality, although, recently, more programs have incorporated measures of efficiency. Many of the quality measures are process measures—that is, they evaluate actions taken by providers, and they tend to measure the proportion of patients in a certain risk group who received some specific type of evidence-based care (e.g., proportion of women ages 52–69 who got a mammogram in the past two years). The measures can be computed from such sources as administrative data, electronic health records, and medical charts. Cost depends on data infrastructure, and auditing is often in place to avoid gaming and cherry-picking patients. The measures might or might not be made available to patients, as well, in which case the information must be useful and understandable to patients.

Similarly, the reward structures of PBAS programs in health care vary widely, from the target of the incentives (physician, medical groups, or hospitals) to the amount of money at risk (varying from $500 to $5,000 per doctor for most programs in the United States to almost

---

[5] P4R legislation was part of the Medicare Prescription Drug Improvement and Modernization Act of 2003 (Public Law 108-173, Medicare Prescription Drug Improvement and Modernization Act of 2003, December 8, 2003), which established the Reporting Hospital Quality Data for Annual Payment Update program and the Physician Quality Reporting Initiative.

$40,000 in the UK program). Such programs are usually structured around meeting specific performance thresholds, but these thresholds can be absolute or relative to other providers. Some programs also pay for improvement. Paying for improvement motivates low performers to improve rather than simply rewarding high performers. The source of the incentive money can be existing funds (so the program is budget-neutral, in which case poor performers might be penalized) or new money (paying out bonuses in addition to existing reimbursement to the successful performers). Since variation in the measures often has some random component (or, in some cases, depends in part on patient behavior), issues of fairness often arise, and some physicians are unwilling to participate in such programs because of the risk. The frequency of the incentive payments (e.g., quarterly, annually) also might have an impact on the effectiveness of PBAS programs, as more-frequent payments might be more salient to providers and thus motivate more-persistent gains in performance.

Despite the popularity of PBAS programs in health care, only a handful of studies have rigorously evaluated their impact. Since many programs in the early stages of PBASs were small in scale, many studies have found only marginal impacts if they found any impact at all. Due to data limitations, these studies have tended to focus on changes in rewarded performance measures only, as opposed to unrewarded measures, which might decrease if providers respond to PBAS incentives by multitasking or teaching to the test (as they do in education). So far, no study has shown PBASs to result in a notable disruption in care. While it is known that design features matter, existing studies do not provide information on the impact of various design features (e.g., number of measures, payment structure, target of the incentives) in any intervention's success or failure.

Public Health Emergency Preparedness

PHEP involves efforts to prevent, protect against, quickly respond to, and recover from large-scale health emergencies, including bioterrorism, naturally occurring disease outbreaks, and natural disasters. Primary legal responsibility for PHEP (as with other aspects of public health) lies with state health departments, which delegate varying degrees of responsibility to local health departments. While PHEP efforts are typically coordinated and led by governmental public health agencies, PHEP also requires active involvement by health-care systems, emergency management, law enforcement, communities, and individuals.

Until recently, the federal role in PHEP was limited largely to providing assistance and coordination during large-scale incidents that stretched state and local capabilities. During the late 1990s, increasing concern about the threat of weapons of mass destruction led to a small federal effort to build state and local ability to prepare for large-scale public health emergencies. That effort grew considerably after September 11, 2001, and the anthrax attacks of October 2001. A survey by the National Association of County and City Health Officials (NACCHO)[6] estimates that 41 percent of local health departments receive all of their PHEP funding from federal sources, while another 40 percent get more than three-fourths of their funding from federal sources.

The two most important federal PHEP programs focus on hospital preparedness (the U.S. Department of Health and Human Services [HHS] Hospital Preparedness Program) and all-hazards public health preparedness (CDC PHEP cooperative agreement). Although the 2002 National Strategy for Homeland Security[7] required that these and other programs create performance measures to evaluate progress, until recently, there were no clearly defined consequences associated with them. The Pandemic and All-Hazards Preparedness Act (PAHPA)[8] clarified those consequences by requiring that HHS, as of

---

[6] National Association of County and City Health Officials, *Federal Funding for Public Health Emergency Preparedness: Implications and Ongoing Issues for Local Health Departments*, Washington, D.C., August 1, 2007.

[7] Office of Homeland Security, *National Strategy for Homeland Security*, Washington, D.C., July 2002. As of June 14, 2010: http://purl.access.gpo.gov/GPO/LPS20641

[8] Public Law 109-417, Pandemic and All-Hazards Preparedness Act, December 20, 2006. As of June 7, 2010: http://frwebgate.access.gpo.gov/cgi-bin/getdoc.cgi?dbname=109_cong_bills&docid=f:s3678enr.txt.pdf

2009, withhold federal funding for failure to meet performance benchmarks. The remainder of this summary focuses on the PHEP cooperative agreement.

The PHEP cooperative agreement requires grantees (including the 50 states, four separately funded large cities, and eight territories) to report data on performance metrics for two program areas: (1) mass medical countermeasure delivery and (2) all other aspects of PHEP. Early metrics focused on infrastructure (e.g., plans, personnel, and equipment), but, more recently, the cooperative agreement has utilized an increasing number of drill-based metrics for assessing operational capabilities (i.e., whether grantees can use infrastructure to complete operational tasks). For instance, a performance metric for the 2009 grant year assesses the amount of time required to notify key incident management staff of the need to report for duty.

Currently, countermeasure delivery is assessed through an extensive written assessment plus five drill-based metrics (grantees must report on three). There are 14 metrics for the remainder of PHEP, focusing on both infrastructure and operational capabilities. Some, but not all, of these metrics are not associated with clear consequences. With the exception of the written assessment on countermeasure delivery (which is administered during site visits by CDC staff), data collection relies on grantee self-reports. While federal data-reporting requirements have applied only to the (mostly state-level) grantees, many states have chosen to require their local grantees to provide data on state-level performance measures before releasing the funds to the local level.

Under the PAHPA legislation, in 2010, CDC must begin withholding funds for failure to meet performance benchmarks. Initially, these benchmarks are linked to a subset of measures that focus on infrastructure and completion of (but not performance on) operational assessments, but, in future years, it is expected that funding will be tied to *levels* of operational performance. States or other grantees failing to meet a benchmark for one year lose 10 percent of their funding. The penalty increases to 15 percent for failure during two consecutive years, 20 percent for three consecutive years, and 25 percent for four consecutive years. HHS might reduce or waive penalties for mitigating conditions, and funds withheld are allocated to hospital preparedness activities within the same jurisdiction. (It should be noted that total budget for the cooperative agreement decreased more than 25 percent in real terms between 2007 and 2009, from $767 million to $609 million).

There are also numerous anecdotes about poor performance ratings on mass medical countermeasure delivery being used by state and local policymakers to justify replacement of key PHEP personnel, thus adding another potential set of consequences associated with the measures.

It is too early to assess the impact of performance-based accountability on PHEP. Nonetheless, there are numerous and widespread anecdotes suggesting that the relatively strong emphasis on performance measurement for mass medical countermeasure delivery has led state and local health departments to invest in those capabilities at the expense of other capabilities. Moreover, the NACCHO survey noted earlier suggests that the threat of funding cuts (on top of those sustained during recent years) are leading local health departments to scale back on preparedness activities.

Transportation

The surface transportation (highway and transit) sector consists of public agencies at all levels of government along with a wide range of private actors. Federal, state, and local governments, in varying degrees, are largely responsible for activities, such as setting policies, raising and distributing revenue, planning and developing projects, and maintaining and operating existing infrastructure. The private sector manufactures personal, commercial, and transit vehicles, and private firms might also contract for such activities as building or maintaining highways or operating transit services.

Performance measurement has a long tradition in the transportation sector, and literally thousands of performance metrics have been developed or discussed. Most commonly, however, performance metrics are used to inform policy and planning decisions. Examples in which performance measures are used to enforce greater accountability are the exception rather than the rule.

PBASs are of growing interest in the field of transportation planning and policy. Federal legislation is expected to be enacted in 2010 that will renew the national transportation-funding program for the following six years. Many politicians, interest groups, and scholars are advocating that familiar formulas by which federal funds are distributed to states for particular programs be replaced by funding arrangements that are "performance-based."[9] Thus far, many state and federal programs purport to measure and report on the performance of the transportation system, but relatively few include any sort of accountability requirements. Current debates suggest that funding should, in the future, be tied more directly to measures of the attainment of major programmatic objectives, such as improved mobility, increased accessibility, and congestion reduction, yet it is not clear that consensus can be reached on approaches by which to measure the attainment of these objectives. For this study, we were unable to find transportation programs that incorporated PBASs, but several specific PBASs were identified within or related to transportation. These were, in general, narrower in scope than some of the pending proposals. For example, in this study, we included examination of road construction contracts that provide bonuses for early completion of a road project and penalties for late project delivery. We also looked at penalties imposed on regions under the CAA amendments when their regional transportation plans failed to result in specified targets for the reduction of air pollutant emissions. Also included was the CAFE program of the federal government, which financially penalizes automobile manufacturers that fail to achieve improvements in fuel economy in pursuit of environmental goals. A fourth transportation-related PBAS is an attempt to reward financially public transit systems that increase their daily patronage in relation to other transit systems. While these four examples cannot, even when taken together, suggest how a more integrated PBAS might work in the field of transportation, they provide many lessons that should influence the design of such a system over the coming few years.

---

[9] National Transportation Policy Project, *Performance Driven: A New Vision for U.S. Transportation Policy*, Washington, D.C.: Bipartisan Policy Center, June 9, 2009.

A+B Highway Construction Contracting Overview

State and local governments often contract with private firms for road construction activities. Traditionally, contracts have been awarded to the firm offering the lowest bid. Some states have adopted performance-based contracting, which is referred to by contractors as A+B contracting because the incentives are enumerated in a section of the contract (part B) that follows the basic contracting language. Under such an incentive-based contract, both the financial cost and the time to complete the project are included in the contract; part A specifies the financial cost, while part B provides rewards for early completion and penalties for late completion. This innovation was motivated by the fact that construction activities create or exacerbate traffic delays. Speeding up project delivery will therefore reduce public costs—in terms of wasted time and fuel—associated with road construction. A+B contracting represents a shift in emphasis from lowest agency cost to best overall public value. Because most highway construction is funded by states (sometimes using federal funds), the gradual shift to A+B contracting has required enabling federal and state policy frameworks.

The principal metric is the time required to complete construction. Contractors are also held to various design and engineering standards, but such standards are not unique to A+B contracting.

A+B contracting relies on financial rewards or sanctions to the construction firm to encourage faster delivery, though the specific form of the incentive can vary depending on how the contract is implemented. In some cases, both time and cost are specified in the bid, but the award price is reduced if the contractor is late in delivering the project. In other cases, only the cost is specified within the bid, but the contractor receives additional bonuses if the project is delivered earlier than the target delivery date. In either case, the size of the bonus or penalty is a function of the number of days that the project is ahead of or behind schedule.

A+B contracting has proven quite successful in reducing the time to complete projects when compared with traditional lowest-bid contracting, and there are many examples in which total construction time has been reduced by more than 50 percent. Provided that the daily bonuses or penalties for early or late delivery are commensurate with the costs, in wasted time and fuel, of construction-related traffic congestion delays, A+B contracting appears to be an effective strategy for minimizing the net social cost of highway construction activities.

Clean Air Act Conformity Requirement Overview

Under the CAA Extension of 1970[10] and subsequent CAA Amendments of 1977[11] and 1990,[12] the U.S. Environmental Protection Agency (EPA) sets ambient air quality standards for several criteria pollutants, including carbon monoxide, nitrogen dioxide, ground-level ozone, sulfur dioxide, fine particulate matter, and lead. Metropolitan regions failing to meet one or more of the EPA criteria-pollutant standards are designated as nonattainment areas. States with nonattainment areas must develop a state implementation plan (SIP) demonstrating how they will achieve compliance with EPA standards by a certain date. Because automobiles and trucks—described as mobile sources—represent a major source of certain pollutants, SIPs often include strategies for reducing mobile-source emissions within each nonattainment area. To strengthen this link, the CAA Amendments of 1990 specified that federal transportation funds be withheld from nonattainment areas that adopt transportation investment plans likely to prevent air quality compliance within the required timeframe.

The initial determination of compliance with EPA's ambient air quality standards is based on sampling the average concentration of the regulated pollutants at different locations over different time intervals. Once an area is found to be in nonattainment, the emphasis shifts to an exercise in forecasting whether the strategies outlined in the SIP, including mobile-source emission-reduction measures, will be sufficient to achieve compliance by the specified target date. From the transportation perspective, a key requirement is to ensure that the planned investments specified in regional transportation plans, such as highway investments, do not undermine the mobile-source emission-reduction targets specified in the SIP. In addition to linking federal

---

[10] Public Law 91-604, Clean Air Act Extension of 1970, December 31, 1970.

[11] Public Law 95-95, Clean Air Act Amendments of 1977, August 8, 1977.

[12] Public Law 101-549, Clean Air Act Amendments of 1990, November 15, 1990.

transportation funding with air quality compliance efforts, the 1990 CAA Amendments also required that the transportation and emission models used by nonattainment areas be more accurate than in previous years, including such features as travel projections by time of day, congestion levels, vehicle speeds, and the interaction of land use and accessibility with travel demand. In effect, the more-accurate modeling requirements make it more difficult to demonstrate compliance, but the results can also be viewed with greater confidence.

The main incentive for complying with EPA's air quality regulations, or, in the case of nonattainment areas, making progress toward compliance, is access to federal transportation dollars. Because large urban regions might receive hundred of millions of dollars per year in federal funding, this is a powerful incentive. Since 1997, conformity lapses (failure to demonstrate progress toward compliance) have occurred in at least 63 areas across 29 states. Most of these areas have returned to conformity quickly and received deferred federal funding without major effects on their transportation program. Five areas, however, had to make significant changes to their transportation plans in order to resolve a conformity lapse. In the most extreme example, the Atlanta region had to strip out the majority of its planned highway expansion projects in order to qualify for about $700 million in federal transportation support.

The success of tying federal transportation funding to compliance with EPA's ambient air quality standards can be viewed as mixed. While air quality has generally improved in the past several decades, there are still many nonattainment areas across the United States. Based on EPA[13] data, in 1992, when federal transportation funding was first linked to conformity, 199 metropolitan areas (out of 340 areas in total), representing a combined population of close to 100 million residents, were classified as nonattainment for one or more criteria pollutants. By 2003, the number had dropped to 100 areas with a total population of 34 million. In 2004 and 2005, after new EPA stan-

---

[13] U.S. Environmental Protection Agency, "The Green Book Nonattainment Areas for Criteria Pollutants," last updated June 16, 2010. As of June 22, 2010: http://epa.gov/airquality/greenbk/

dards related to ozone and fine particulate matter came into force, the number of nonattainment areas jumped to 201, representing around 190 million residents. By 2008, however, the number of nonattainment areas had declined to about 140, with a combined population of 178 million. In short, the past two decades have witnessed slow but steady improvement toward attainment of air quality goals; while the number of nonattainment areas increased in 2004 and 2005, this was due to the application of two additional demanding standards.

Several additional factors complicate the assessment. First, many of the recent improvements in air quality can be attributed to innovations in vehicle emission control technology rather than transportation infrastructure planning and investment. At the same time, mobile sources are not solely responsible for air quality problems; stationary sources (e.g., factories or refineries) also emit harmful pollutants, so failure to achieve compliance is not just a function of transportation planning. What we can say for certain is that the link to federal funding has been sufficient to induce some regions, such as Atlanta, to cancel infrastructure investments likely to further exacerbate air quality challenges.

Corporate Average Fuel Economy Standards Overview

Introduced with the Energy Policy and Conservation Act (EPCA)[14] in response to the oil shocks of 1973–1974, CAFE standards require that automobile manufacturers achieve a minimum level of fuel economy for the fleet of vehicles sold each year in the United States. Manufacturers failing to meet the standards are subject to significant fines. Separate CAFE standards are applied to passenger cars and light trucks (e.g., minivans, sport-utility vehicles [SUVs], and pickup trucks), with the former being more stringent. Passenger-car standards were first enforced in 1978, and light-truck standards in 1979. During the 1980s and early 1990s, the standards were made more demanding with some regularity, but, in recent years, the standards have been allowed to stagnate. The passenger-car standard of 27.5 miles per gallon (mpg), for example, has remained constant since 1990, while the light-truck stan-

---

[14] Public Law 94-163, Energy Policy and Conservation Act, December 22, 1975.

dard of 20.7 mpg has not been increased since 1996. With growing concern over such issues as climate change, energy security, and fuel price volatility, however, there has been a renewed interest in more-stringent fuel economy standards. In response to increased public pressure, Congress passed the Energy Independence and Security Act of 2007,[15] which requires that auto manufacturers once again begin to increase the average fuel economy of their fleets. The new regulations take effect in model year 2011 and will culminate in a fleetwide average of 35 mpg by 2020.

Under CAFE regulations, EPA is responsible for rating the fuel economy for each vehicle model that a manufacturer produces, using a standardized test procedure on new vehicles taken at random from assembly lines. Manufacturers are then judged according to the sales-weighted fuel economy of the fleet of vehicles they sell in the United States each year, based on a set of assumptions regarding typical driving patterns. Fleet fuel-economy measures are calculated separately for passenger cars and light trucks.

If the average fuel economy of a manufacturer's passenger-car or light-truck fleet fails to meet the corresponding CAFE standard, the manufacturer must pay a penalty of $5.50 for each 0.1-mpg shortfall multiplied by the number of vehicles produced for the U.S. market. Manufacturers earn CAFE credits in years when they exceed the standard, which can be applied to offset shortfalls in the preceding or following three years. The rationale for such credits is to ensure that manufacturers are penalized only for persistent failure to meet requirements, not for temporary noncompliance due to anomalous market conditions in any specific year. The threat of sanctions appears to be generally effective, as most manufacturers, including the major U.S. and Japanese firms, consistently meet CAFE standards. Some high-end producers, however, such as BMW, Daimler, Ferrari, Porsche, and Maserati, choose to pay the fines rather than trying to meet the CAFE requirements.

---

[15] Public Law 110-140, Energy Independence and Security Act of 2007, December 19, 2007. As of June 14, 2010: http://frwebgate.access.gpo.gov/cgi-bin/getdoc.cgi?dbname=110_cong_public_laws&docid=f:publ140.110

CAFE standards are generally recognized as having had a positive effect on reducing motor fuel consumption in the United States. That said, the CAFE approach to fuel economy remains controversial for several reasons:

- A common strategy for improving vehicle fuel economy is to reduce vehicle weight. Safety proponents have argued that lighter cars increase the risk of crash fatalities, though other studies suggest that vehicle design and quality are stronger determinants of safety than vehicle weight.
- Economists have suggested that simply taxing fuel consumption, though perhaps more politically challenging, would be a far more-efficient approach for stimulating the production and consumption of more fuel-efficient vehicles.
- The decoupling of light-truck and passenger-vehicle mileage standards, when combined with significant growth in the market share for light trucks in the past several decades, has undermined the fleetwide improvement in fuel economy that might otherwise have been achieved.

Transit Subsidy Formula Allocation Overview

Congress established the National Transit Database (NTD) as the primary source for information and statistics on U.S. transit systems. The database was intended to collect and publish data that individual transit systems could use for service planning and that federal, state, and local governments could use for transit investment decisionmaking. More than 660 transit providers in urbanized areas currently report to the NTD through a standardized reporting system. Each year, NTD performance data are used to apportion more than $5 billion of Federal Transit Administration (FTA) funds to transit agencies in urbanized areas, mostly for *capital* projects. State and regional transportation agencies, however, support more than 95 percent of transit *operating* costs, and the uses of NTD data for subsidy allocation vary widely from state to state.

An extensive body of research dating back to the late 1970s evaluates and establishes measures of transit service effectiveness, efficiency, and productivity. These studies examine the appropriateness and uses of various performance measures (such as cost efficiency, cost-effectiveness, service utilization, vehicle utilization, quality of service, labor productivity, and coverage) and performance indicators (e.g., cost per mile, cost per passenger trip, passenger trips per vehicle mile, miles per vehicle, average speed, passenger trips per employee, vehicle miles per capita). These studies also examine the use of nontraditional indicators that are not collected by the NTD. Most research finds general consensus among transit agencies and experts that funding and investment decisions should incorporate a combination of performance indicators when comparing peer groups and that such indicators should be consistent with transit agencies' goals. However, there are strong disagreements about which measures to use and how to combine them into a composite index.

Most states allocate operating subsidies based on a formula process; some states include performance-based measures in these formulas, while the majority use only non–performance-based measures (such as level of local financial match, or service population). Very few states, if any, use wholly performance-based measures and procedures. Studies have identified three general trends in the use of performance measures for transit funding allocation: When performance measures are used, they are (1) combined with nonperformance measures in a composite index, (2) used to determine an incentive level of funding above a baseline set by non–performance-based measures, or (3) eventually eliminated completely from any formula allocation procedures.

For example, following a six-year implementation process, transit operators in Indiana now are categorized into four peer groups based on scale and scope of services and agency size. Funding is then allocated within each of the four peer groups based on a formula that provides equal weight to passengers per operating expense, miles per operating expense, and locally derived income per operating expense. The data used are calculated on a three-year rolling average to enhance funding stability and predictability. Other states that currently use performance measures in transit funding include Florida, Iowa, Ohio, New York, North Carolina, Pennsylvania, Missouri, and California. Texas created a formula based on demographic and performance data in 1989 but abandoned it in 1994; it now allocates based on financial need.

There has been little evaluation of whether the use of performance measures in transit funding allocation has resulted in service-delivery improvements. However, some studies have examined reasons that state and regional governments have followed the general trend of separating performance measurement from funding. Findings suggest that (1) formulas have not produced revenue or funding changes significant enough to affect service-delivery behaviors, especially when performance measures are used to determine an incentive level, rather than a base level of funding; (2) philosophical debates arise about whether to penalize agencies most in need; (3) the political process of funding allocation tends to favor distributional equity over operational goals; (4) transit satisfies a broad-based set of goals, many of which cannot be captured in performance measures; (5) lag time between reporting and allocation decisions make the PBAS difficult to administer; and (6) the zero-sum nature of limited transit funding is not likely to garner support for a PBAS that rewards some operators at the expense of others.